THE COMPLETE CANCER RECIPE COOKBOOK

FOOD RECIPES THAT CAN HELP DESTROY CANCER CELLS IN THE BODY.

Rose Walter

INTRODUCTION

Welcome to a culinary voyage dedicated to both indulgence and well-being. In a world where nutrition plays a pivotal role in our health, we present a recipe designed with a purpose – to harness the natural properties of ingredients believed to combat cancer cells within the body. As we delve into the art of cooking, our focus extends beyond flavor, venturing into the realm of potential health benefits. This recipe is a symphony of carefully chosen components, each renowned for its alleged capacity to support the body's defenses against cancer. From antioxidant-rich vegetables to anti-inflammatory spices, every element is a deliberate addition aimed at creating a dish that not only tantalizes the taste buds but also contributes to a proactive approach to health.

Science suggests that certain foods possess compounds with anti-cancer properties, and this culinary creation endeavors to bring them together in a delightful amalgamation. Join us in this culinary exploration, where the joy of eating is fused with a commitment to nurturing your body, one mouthwatering bite at a time. Let's savor the flavors of a recipe that aspires to be more than just a meal – a potential ally in the ongoing quest for well-being.

Are you wondering how to prepare delectable dishes that may help ward off cancer? Nutritious meals with some of the most potent anti-cancer foods—such as blueberries, raspberries, sweet potatoes, asparagus, avocados, carrots, beets, and more—are included in this recipe collection. The dishes in this collection, which combat cancer, not only highlight foods high in anti-cancer nutrients, but also have low nitrate levels, a low glycemic index, and minimal to no animal fat. Before diving into cancer-fighting recipes.

CHAPTER 1

RECIPES FOR CANCER PREVENTION DISHES.(MAIN MEAL)

Are you looking for creative soup recipes that are perfect for those seeking natural cancer prevention methods? There's nowhere else to look! This area offers a rainbow of anti-cancer recipes made with foods that are rich in nutrients that fight cancer, like beta-carotene, astaxanthin, glutathione, and vitamin C.

Asparagus with Quince Jam and Walnuts

Ingredients

Two pounds of washed and trimmed asparagus spears

Two tsp freshly grated ginger

Two tablespoons of quince jam

Two tablespoons pure olive oil

One teaspoon of lemon juice

3 tbsp chopped walnuts

To taste, add salt and freshly ground black pepper.

Guidelines

Boil water in a steamer to prepare it. Add asparagus, cover, and steam for three to five minutes, or until tender and crisp. After cooking, move the asparagus to a serving dish.

Combine the ginger, quince jam, lemon juice, olive oil, salt, and pepper in a small bowl. Drizzle over the asparagus. Add chopped walnuts on top.

Shrimp and Mushroom Risotto

Ingredients

Three tablespoons of olive oil

1/4 pound of cleaned, stemmed, and chopped cremini mushrooms

1/4 pound of peeled and deveined prawns

one minced clove of garlic

One onion, chopped finely

One and a third cups of raw long-grain brown rice

4 1/4 cup broth made with vegetables

3 tablespoons chopped fresh chives

1/4 pound of thawed frozen peas

Add pepper and salt.

Guidelines

Heat 2 tablespoons of olive oil in a big pot. Season with salt and pepper and add the prawns and mushrooms. Cook for three to five minutes, tossing frequently, or until prawns are cooked through. Place on a platter and reserve.

In the same pot, add minced onion and garlic and heat another tablespoon of olive oil. Let onions sauté for a few minutes, or until they start to become transparent.Stir the rice and continue cooking for a few minutes.

Pour in a half-cup of broth. Cook until nearly all of the broth is absorbed, stirring from time to time. Once all of the broth has been used and the rice is almost cooked, add another half cup of broth every time the liquid is absorbed (use water if you run out of broth towards the end).

Add the sautéed prawns, mushrooms and peas. Cook, stirring frequently, for a few minutes. To taste, add salt and pepper for seasoning. Serve right away after transferring to serving plates.

Arugula, Avocado and Tomato

Ingredients

Three cups of new, washed rocket leaves

Two cups of halved cherry tomatoes

1/4 cup chopped sun-dried tomatoes

Two teaspoons pure olive oil

One-third cup balsamic vinegar

Two tiny avocados, cut, pitted, and peeled

Guidelines

Add the rocket, cherry tomatoes, sun-dried tomatoes, olive oil and vinegar to a big plastic dish that fits tight on a lid. Toss well.

Transfer to plates, then place a few avocado slices on top of each serving.

Beet and Carrot Salad with Ginger

Ingredients

half a cup of raw, grated, peeled beets

Grated half a cup of organic carrots

Two tablespoons of apple juice

One tablespoon pure olive oil

1 tsp finely chopped fresh ginger

1/8 teaspoon sea salt

Guidelines

In a small bowl, mix grated carrots and beets.

In a separate bowl, combine the apple juice, olive oil, salt, and ginger; sprinkle over the salad mixture. Gently toss. Have fun!

Grandma's Chicken Soups

Ingredients:

1 whole chicken

8 cups chicken broth

3 carrots,

 3 celery stalks,

1 onion,

 3 cloves garlic,

1 cup chopped potatoes

1 cup chopped leeks

1 teaspoon dried thyme

1 bay leaf

Salt and pepper to taste Fresh parsley for garnish

Instructions:

In a large pot, combine the chicken pieces and chicken broth. Bring to a boil, then reduce the heat and simmer for 30 minutes, skimming any foam that rises to the surface.

Add carrots, celery, onion, garlic, potatoes, leeks, thyme, bay leaf, salt, and pepper to the pot. Simmer for an additional 30-40 minutes until the vegetables are tender and the chicken is cooked through.

Remove the chicken pieces from the soup, shred the meat, and return it to the pot.

Taste the soup and adjust seasoning if needed. Remove the bay leaf.

Serve the chicken soup hot, garnished with fresh parsley.

Enjoy the comforting flavors of grandma's chicken soup!

Chicken Soup with Rice and Broccoli

Ingredients

Four cups of low-sodium, fat-free chicken broth

One little onion, finely sliced

1 1/2 cups of florets of broccoli

two little ribs chopped organic celery

Half a cup of rinsed short grain brown rice and two tiny carrots

Two cups of cooked, chopped skinless chicken

Guidelines

Soak rice in cold water from 15 minutes to one hour. Cooking time will be shortened as a result.

Place broth in a large pot and bring to a boil. Add veggies and rice that has been presoaked. Once the rice is soft, turn down the heat to low, cover, and cook it while stirring now and then.

Simmer for 3–4 minutes after adding the prepared chicken.

Romaine and Smoked Salmon Salad

Ingredients

One tiny organic head of romaine lettuce

Five ounces of thinly sliced smoked salmon

two chopped tomatoes

4 radishes, 1 organic carrot, 1 peeled and chopped cucumber, and 1 carrot sliced diagonally

Juice from one-half lemon

One teaspoon freshly peeled and chopped ginger root

One tablespoon of canola oil

Guidelines

Divide the romaine lettuce into two dishes. Top with salmon, tomatoes, radishes, carrots, and cucumber.

In a firmly closed container, shake together the lemon juice, canola oil, and minced ginger. Dollop on salad

CHAPTER 2

Tangy Tomato Soup with Basil.

Ingredients

Three big cloves of garlic

3 oz of sliced, peeled shallots

One tablespoon of olive oil

One 14 1/2-oz can of undrained stewed tomatoes

Half a cup of chicken broth

Apple cider vinegar, 1/2 teaspoon

One-fourth teaspoon salt

A tiny pinch of finely powdered red pepper

Chop 2 tablespoons of fresh basil

Guideline

Place the peeled and crushed garlic aside. The health benefits of crushed or minced garlic are enhanced when it is left for at least five to ten minutes after crushing.

While the health-promoting compounds in the crushed garlic are developing, place the shallots, tomatoes, apple cider vinegar, and chicken broth in a food processor or blender and mix until smooth.

In a big, nonstick saucepan, warm up the olive oil over medium heat. Stir continuously for about 30 seconds after adding the garlic.

Barley Soup with Beans and Basil

Ingredients:

1/4 cup finely sliced yellow onion

One little carrot, chopped and

One rib celery, cut finely

One tablespoon of virgin olive oil

Five cups of vegetable stock

half a cup cooked pearled barley

half a cup of cooked white beans

one-fourth cup of canned tomatoes

four minced garlic cloves

3 tablespoons chopped fresh basil

1/2 tsp of rosemary, dry

To taste, add salt and pepper.

Guidelines

Simmer onion in olive oil in a soup pot over medium
heat for 4–5 minutes, or until tender. Add the carrots and
celery. Simmer for three minutes or so.

Once added, bring the vegetable broth to a boil. Simmer the soup until the celery and carrots are soft.

Stir in the tinned tomatoes, cooked beans, garlic, rosemary, and cooked barley. Simmer for an additional minute or two.

Add little salt and pepper .

Curried Sweet Potato Soup

Ingredients

One tablespoon canola oil

One large yellow onion, diced coarsely

1 crushed garlic clove and 2 tsp curry powder

1 and a half pounds of peeled and chopped sweet potatoes (pink, orange, or yellow) and a half-inch piece of fresh ginger

3 cups of vegetable broth with minimal sodium

Parsley, chopped, as a garnish

Heat oil in a medium saucepan over medium heat. Stir continuously for approximately 30 seconds after adding the curry powder and garlic.

Over medium-high heat, add the sweet potatoes, onion, ginger, and broth; bring to a boil. After lowering the heat to medium-low, simmer the sweet potatoes for 20 to 25 minutes, or until they are easily pierced with a fork.

Blend soup until smooth using an immersion hand blender or a blender.

Stir-Fried Asparagus with Quinoa Noodles

Ingredients:

 2 bunches of asparagus, chopped into bite-sized pieces after washing and trimming.

One tablespoon of olive oil

3 tsp finely chopped fresh ginger

Two slivered cloves of garlic

One tablespoon of soy sauce

Half a tablespoon of sugar

3.25 tablespoons vegetable stock

Dried quinoa noodles, 12 oz.

Guidelines

In a pan with heated oil, stir-fry the ginger and garlic for one or two minutes before adding the asparagus.

Pour the tiny bowl's contents—soy sauce, sugar, and stock—over the asparagus. Simmer for three to five minutes, or until asparagus is tender.

Noodles should be cooked as per the instructions on the package and served with stir-fried asparagus.

Carrot and Avocado Salad

Ingredients

One big avocado, chopped, pitted, and peeled

4 medium-sized carrots, shredded and peel

Balsamic vinegar dash

Sunflower seeds, flavor-infused

To taste, add salt and freshly ground pepper.

Guidelines

In a medium salad bowl, mix grated carrots and avocado. Add balsamic vinegar, salt, pepper, and sunflower seeds.

Before serving, cover and chill for at least 20 minutes.

Tomato, Cucumber and Red Onion Salad

Ingredients

Two large cucumbers, cut finely after peeling

three big tomatoes, roughly sliced

2.3 cups finely sliced red onion

one-third cup balsamic vinegar

A half-tsp white sugar

Turmeric, three tablespoons of extra virgin

To taste, add salt and pepper.

For garnish, use fresh mint or basil leaves (optional).

Guidelines

Combine all the ingredients in a big basin that can be covered. To combine, cover and shake.

Add pepper and salt for seasoning.

Super-Nutritious Broccoli Salad with Apples and Cranberries

Rich in a variety of nutrients, this low-GI broccoli salad with apples and cranberries is low in fat and calories.

Ingredients

Fresh broccoli florets in four cups

Dried cranberries, half a cup

half a cup of sunflower seeds

Three apples that are organic

1/4 cup finely sliced red onion

One cup of plain, low-fat yoghurt infused with probiotics

Two tablespoons Dijon mustard

1/4 cup of honey

Guidelines

In a large serving bowl, combine broccoli florets, diced apples, chopped onion, sunflower seeds, and dried cranberries. In a small bowl, blend together yoghurt, mustard, and honey.

Breakfast Recipes with Cancer-Fighting Potential

Are you trying to come up with mouthwatering breakfast recipes that can also help fight cancer? This portion of our Guide to Combating Cancer is brimming with recipes for breakfast foods that use foods like blueberries, carrots, oats, and red grapes that may help fight cancer.

But before you let your inner chef out and try out these breakfast recipes, it could be a good idea to read this guide's sections on diet (Best Diet Tips for Cancer Prevention) and food (Best Foods for Fighting Cancer) to learn more about how your diet affects your risk of developing cancer.

Dairy-Free Blueberry Muesli

Ingredients

1 50 ml of rolled oats

Half a cup of chopped walnuts

Chopped 1/2 cup dry apples; 2 tsp ground cinnamon

Two cups of wild, ideally blueberries

three tablespoons of brown sugar

Serve apple juice.

Instructions

Turn the oven on to 325°F, or 160°C on gas 3.

Combine sugar, cinnamon, and oats in a bowl. Using a nonstick baking tray, evenly distribute the ingredients.

For around ten minutes, toast the oat mixture in a preheated oven, stirring periodically. As the mixture toasts, keep a close eye on it because it can burn easily.

Take out of the oven and leave to cool. Transfer into a spacious basin, then mix in chopped walnuts and dehydrated apples.

Spoon mixture into serving dishes; garnish with blueberries. Accompany with a glass of apple juice.

Oat and Buckwheat Muesli with Pears and Grapes.

Ingredients:

One and a half cups of rolled oats

Half a cup of puffy buckwheat

1/4 cup chopped dry apples; 2 tsp ground cinnamon

One cup of chopped organic pears

1 cup red grapes, cut in half; 3 tablespoons brown sugar

To serve, rice milk

Guidelines

Set oven temperature to 325°F (160°C, gas 3).

Oats should be uniformly spread out onto a nonstick baking tray and toasted for about ten minutes, stirring periodically, in a preheated oven. When toasting oats, keep a tight eye on them because they can burn easily.

Take it out of the oven and let it cool. Transfer into a large glass or ceramic bowl and top with water. Soak for the entire night in the refrigerator.

To soaked oats, add brown sugar, cinnamon, puffed buckwheat, and dried apples. Mix thoroughly.

Pour mixture into serving dishes, then add pears and grapes on top. Accompany with rice water.

Oat and Wheat Germ Muesli with Apples

Ingredients:

1 1/2 cups rolled oats, uncooked or toasted

Half a cup wheat germ (where to get it)

two tsp of cinnamon powder

1 1/2 cups chopped organic apples

Two tablespoons of brown sugar

Probiotic-infused organic yoghurt to be served

Guidelines

Set oven temperature to 325°F (160°C, gas 3).

In a bowl, combine the oats, sugar, and cinnamon. Evenly spread the mixture onto a baking tray that is nonstick.

Oat mixture should be toasty for about ten minutes in a hot oven, stirring periodically. When toasting, keep a tight eye on the mixture because it might burn easily.

Take it out of the oven and let it cool. Transfer to a sizable bowl and mix in the wheat germ.

Spoon mixture into serving bowls; garnish with raspberries and apples. Accompany with yoghurt.

Original Bircher Muesli

Ingredients:

1 tablespoon rolled oats

Three tablespoons of water

One tablespoon sweetened condensed milk
two teaspoons of lemon juice

One or two apples, with skin on

1 tablespoon ground hazelnuts or almonds

Guidelines

Blend oats with water and keep chilled for the entire night. Because phytic acid can prevent the absorption of numerous minerals in the intestines, soaking enhances the nutritious value of oats by enabling enzymes to break down and neutralise this substance.

Cut up apples. Add them to the soaked oats along with the lemon juice and sweetened condensed milk. Mix thoroughly.

After that, serve with a dusting of almond or hazelnuts.

Antioxidant Muffins

Ingredients

One cup of flour made from whole wheat

one-third cup of brown sugar

A half-tsp of baking powder

Chopped pecans, 1/3 cup

One-fourth teaspoon salt

One cup of blueberries

one-fourth cup almond milk

One big egg

Guidelines

Set oven temperature to 350°F (177°C, gas 4).

Mix together flour, sugar, pecans, baking powder, and salt. Beat the egg and almond milk together gently in another bowl. Mix the wet and dry ingredients together.

Transfer mixture into paper muffin liners. After baking for thirty to forty minutes, move the muffins to a cooling rack. Warm up and serve.

Carrot Muffins

Ingredients

One egg

One cup rice milk

Four tablespoons of canola oil

Two cups of gluten-free flour, such as quinoa flour

One teaspoon guar gum

One tablespoon of flaxseed meal

3. 1/2 tsp baking powder free of gluten

Half a teaspoon of salt

One teaspoon of cinnamon

One-fourth cup brown sugar

one cup grated organic carrots

one-fourth cup raisins

Guidelines

Set oven temperature to 400°F (200°C, gas mark 6).

Beat the egg, canola oil, and rice milk together. Mix the dry ingredients together in a separate basin.

Mix the liquid ingredients into the dry ingredients just until combined; do not overmix. Stir in the raisins and grated carrots.

Cake should be poured into 12 paper muffin cups, about two thirds full. Bake for 20 minutes.

Ingredients:

QuinoaFresh berries (e.g., blueberries, strawberries)FlaxseedsHoneyChopped nuts (e.g., almonds, walnuts)Optional: A pinch of cinnamon for flavorHerbal tea for taste.

Method

Rinse quinoa, cook with veggies and protein, assemble in a bowl, drizzle with dressing, top with seeds or herbs.

CHAPTER 3

ANTI-CANCER DESSERT RECIPES

Green Tea Mango Blast

Ingredients:

Two cups of diced and peeled mango

One cup of loose leaf green tea

One tablespoon honey

a freshly peeled and finely chopped half-inch piece of fresh ginger

one cup of ice, crushed

In a food processor or blender, combine all ingredients and mix until smooth.

Garnish to taste, and serve with eco-straws of sturdy borosilicate glass, bamboo, or stainless steel.

Flourless Chocolate Cake

A surprise addition to this flourless chocolate cake is black beans! Black beans are high in fibre and protein but low in calories and fat. In addition, dark, unsweetened cocoa powder—the kind of chocolate known for its potent antioxidant qualities—is needed for this recipe.

Ingredients:

One and a half cups of cooked black beans

Four big eggs

One tablespoon of mint essence

One tsp of stevia

5 tablespoons vegetable oil

one-third cup honey

Half a teaspoon of dark, unsweetened cocoa powder

One teaspoon of baking powder

One-half teaspoon baking soda

A dash of salt

fresh mint leaves as a garnish

Guidelines

Set oven temperature to 350°F (177°C, gas 4).

In a blender, process beans, 2 eggs, stevia, oil, honey, and mint extract until fully smooth.

Whisk together the cocoa powder, baking soda, and baking powder.

In a small bowl, beat the remaining two eggs. Thoroughly combine the egg mixture with the bean batter. Add the cocoa powder and beat on high speed until the mixture is smooth.

Fill a 9-inch cake pan with batter, oil it, and bake for 35 to 45 minutes, or until a toothpick inserted into the cake comes out clean.

Low-Fat Apple and Raspberry Crumble

Ingredients:

Five big cooking apples, cut into thin slices

One cup of raspberries

two glasses of apple juice

Two cups of rolled oats

Two tsp margarine or butter

Two tablespoons of brown sugar

Two teaspoons of cinnamon

Half a teaspoon of cloves

Adjust the oven's gas to 350°F.

Put the raspberries and apple slices in a baking dish that has been greased. Drizzle with apple juice.In a medium bowl, combine rolled oats, sugar, and spices. Using your fingertips, cut in butter or margarine until distributed evenly.

Dredge the raspberries and apples in the crumble topping.

Bake in a preheated oven for 45 to 60 minutes. Serve warm or cold.

Whole Wheat Brownies

This whole wheat brownie recipe is a healthy substitute for many other brownie recipes, and these brownies are packed with flavour.

Ingredients:

3 tablespoons low-sodium butter

Half a cup of brown rice syrup

10 tablespoons unsweetened dark cocoa powder

One teaspoon vanilla

two eggs

Half a cup of whole wheat flour

Half a cup of chopped pecans

Guidelines

Melt butter in a medium saucepan over low heat. Blend in chocolate powder and brown rice syrup. Whisk continuously until thoroughly combined.

Take off the heat and mix in the eggs.

Mix thoroughly after adding the pecans, vanilla, and whole wheat flour.

Grease an 8 × 8-inch baking sheet lightly, then add the batter. Remove the toothpick after 30 minutes of baking.

After letting cool, cut into squares.serve.

Rice Pudding with Blueberry Sauce

Ingredients:

One cup of rice, brown basmati

3 cups rice milk, 2 cups water, and 1/2 teaspoon salt

one-third cup of brown sugar

1/2 teaspoon ground cinnamon

One teaspoon potato starch

Instructions:

In a medium saucepan, combine rice, water, and salt; bring to a boil. Turn down the heat to low, cover, and simmer for 45 minutes or until the water is completely absorbed, stirring now and then.

Mix thoroughly after adding the cinnamon, brown sugar, and rice milk. Stirring now and then, cook for another ten minutes.

In a separate bowl, combine potato starch and a few drops of water; stir into rice mixture. Stirring continuously over low heat, the mixture will take about 5 minutes to thicken and achieve pudding-like consistency. Take off the heat.

Move to a spacious bowl,cover, and refrigerate until cold, about 2 hours. Serve with warm blueberry sauce.

Buckwheat Crepes with Prune Compote

Ingredients:

two eggs

1/4 cup rice milk

1/3 cup quinoa flour and 2/3 cup buckwheat flour

One tablespoon canola oil

Half a teaspoon of salt

For frying, use vegetable cooking spray.

Eight ounces of pitted and softened organic dried plums in warm water

one cup of water

One tablespoon of brown sugar

One tablespoon of apple juice

Guidelines

In a medium-sized bowl, beat eggs. Whisk together rice milk, buckwheat flour, quinoa flour, canola oil, and salt thoroughly.

Set a big nonstick skillet on medium heat to get it ready. Apply cooking spray intended for vegetables.

Pour about 1/3 cup of batter into the skillet for the first pancake, then rapidly rotate the skillet to coat the bottom evenly. Cook pancake for one to two minutes over medium-high heat, or until bubbles start to form. Turn over and continue to cook for 30-60 seconds, take out of the skillet.

Once the batter is gone, repeat the previous process.

Put the prunes, apple juice, sugar, and water in a saucepan and bring to a boil to make prune compote. Once the prunes become tender, reduce the heat and simmer for 12 to 15 minutes.

Let prune compote cool for a few minutes, then serve on crepes.

Quinoa Crepes with Applesauce

Ingredients

(1) Half quinoa flour

1 tsp baking soda and 1/2 cup tapioca flour

One teaspoon of cinnamon

two cups of fizzy water

Three tablespoons of canola oil

Three cups of organic, unsalted apple sauce

To taste, cinnamon

Guidelines

Combine cinnamon, baking soda, tapioca flour, and quinoa flour in a medium-sized bowl. Whisk in the oil and water until thoroughly blended.

Set a big nonstick skillet on medium heat to get it ready. Add a few canola oil droplets.
Pour about 1/3 cup of batter into the skillet for the first pancake, then rapidly rotate the skillet to coat the bottom evenly. Cook pancake over medium-high heat till light brown on the bottom. Turn, then quickly cook the other side.

Once the batter is gone, repeat the previous process. Accompany with applesauce.

Scandinavian Blueberry Soup (Blåbärssoppa)

Ingredients

Four cups of blueberries

1/2 cup sugar and 2 cups of water

4 tsp potato flour

Guidelines

Put the water, sugar, and blueberries in a pot and heat until boiling.

Stir potato starch into the blueberry mixture after mixing it with a few drops of cold water. Stir the soup continuously over low heat until it thickens.

Transfer to a platter and serve right away. As an alternative, you might chill the soup in the refrigerator, sprinkle it with sugar, and serve it that way.

Recipes for Anti-Cancer Smoothies and Drinks

Are you keen to discover how to create delicious smoothies and other beverages that meet the nutritional requirements of individuals on an anti-cancer diet? There are a tonne of drink ideas in this section that contain foods that can combat cancer, such as smoothies. It could be a good idea to first peruse the sections on the best foods for fighting cancer and the best diet tips for cancer prevention, which offer more general information about how what you eat and drink can affect your risk of getting cancer, before you let your inner chef loose and try out the incredibly healthful drink recipes below.

Catechin-Rich Ice Tea

Ingredients:

two cups of water

2 1/2 teaspoons of loose green tea leaves (tea bags produce less catechins than loose leaves do)

Three tablespoons of newly squeezed organic lemon juice

Guidelines

Heat the water to a boil. Put the green tea leaves in the teapot and fill it with boiling water. Give it five minutes to steep.

After straining the tea, add the lemon juice (vitamin C rich lemon juice helps the body more readily absorb the green tea's catechins).

Before serving, place in the refrigerator and chill fully.

Serve with sustainable straws made of bamboo, stainless steel, or hard borosilicate glass.

Hot Chocolate with Almond Milk

Ingredients:

Five tablespoons of brown sugar

Three teaspoons of dark, unsweetened cocoa powder

Two glasses of almond milk without sugar

Half a teaspoon vanilla extract

Guidelines

Put the cocoa and sugar into a small pot. Add almond milk and whisk.

Heat over medium heat, stirring all the time, until heated through. Avoid boiling.

Take off the heat and mix in the vanilla. With glass straws, serve hot.

Turmeric-Ginger Mango Smoothie Bowl

Ingredients:

- 1 ripe mango, peeled and chopped
- 1 frozen banana, chopped
- 1 cup spinach leaves
- 1-inch piece of fresh ginger, peeled and grated
- 1 tsp ground turmeric
- 1 cup unsweetened almond milk (or any milk alternative)
- 1 tbsp chia seeds
- 1 tbsp flaxseed meal
- Toppings: sliced strawberries, blueberries, toasted coconut flakes, and pumpkin seeds

Instructions:

1. In a blender, combine the mango, frozen banana, spinach, grated ginger, ground turmeric, almond milk, chia seeds, and flaxseed meal.
2. Blend on high until smooth and creamy.

CONCLUSION

"The Complete Cancer Recipe Cookbook" offers a comprehensive collection of recipes tailored to support individuals dealing with cancer. this cookbook provides a valuable resource for those seeking nourishing meals during their journey. The diverse range of recipes not only caters to different dietary preferences but also emphasizes ingredients known for their potential health benefits. Overall, this cookbook serves as a practical guide, promoting well-balanced and enjoyable culinary choices for individuals navigating the challenges of cancer.